When a Heart Transplant Changes Everything. What Do You Do Next? How Would You Feel?

Here are 15 Steps to guide you through the process of supporting your loved one and yourself.

Hearing that someone you love needs a heart transplant is overwhelming. Fear, uncertainty, and countless questions can take over in an instant.

There's no roadmap for this experience, but you don't have to face it alone. At the core of it all are two powerful forces: unwavering love and unshakable faith.

In her book, *Your Amazing Itty Bitty™ Caregiver's Guide for a Heart Transplant Recipient*, Luann Owens shares her experience and provides you with the tools you need on how to:

- Show up with structure and consistency
- Create a safe, healing home environment
- Support a heart-healthy lifestyle
- Celebrate every milestone
- And so much more!

If you're facing the unexpected, this book will guide you forward one step at a time. Pick up your copy today!

Your Amazing Itty Bitty™ Caregiver's Guide for a Heart Transplant Recipient

15 Key Steps to Supporting Your Loved One and Yourself

Luann DeBiase Owens

Published by Itty Bitty™ Publishing
A subsidiary of S & P Productions, Inc.

Your Amazing Itty Bitty™ Caregiver's Guide for a Heart Transplant Recipient by Luann DeBiase Owens

Printed in the United States of America

Itty Bitty Publishing
311 Main Street, Suite D
El Segundo, CA 90245
(310) 640-8885

ISBN: 978-1-959964-63-6

This book is for educational purposes only.Nothing should be taken as physical or mental health advice, diagnosis, or treatment. Always seek the guidance of a health care professional should you need assistance.

Dedication

I dedicate this book to my husband Jimmy, whose heart and resolve are as strong as a lion's. And to God with deepest gratitude for His grace and for saving my husband's life.

Stop by our Itty Bitty™ website to find interesting information regarding caregiving for transplant patients

www.IttyBittyPublishing.com

Or visit Luann Owens at

http://jimmyowens.com/Luann

Table of Contents

Introduction

I never planned on becoming the caregiver of a heart transplant patient, but life has a way of choosing us before we're ready.

When my husband's heart began to fail, we didn't have a roadmap. No one handed me an instruction manual titled, "Here's Everything You Should Know." What I had instead was love, faith, and determination. If you're holding this book, there's a good chance you're carrying a weight of your own.

This book is for you; these 15 steps will help you understand what lies ahead and give you insight to a whole new world of caring for an organ recipient. There is no information given to you at the start of this journey. This book will give you some insight and help alleviate some of the fear that comes from the unknown of what is an already stressful situation.

Step 1
Shock of Diagnosis

When you first hear that your loved one's heart is failing and a transplant may be necessary, your world shifts instantly. As a caregiver, you are thrown into a situation that feels overwhelming and unfamiliar. Your emotions are valid, and there are steps you can take to regain a sense of control.

1. You may experience shock, fear, anger, or disbelief.
2. Allow yourself to feel.
3. Your emotions are real and normal.
4. Don't push them away; acknowledge them. Process them and move forward.

Ask questions. Doctors often speak in medical terms that can feel overwhelming. As a caregiver, you need clarity. Remember, there are no silly questions when it comes to your loved one's life.

1. Keep a notebook with you to jot down what the doctors say.
2. Repeat their answers back to confirm you understand.
3. Write everything down. The amount of information you receive is impossible to remember.

More About the Shock of Diagnosis

At first, everything seems confusing. But knowledge is power. The more you understand about how a transplant works, the less frightening it will seem.

- Work closely with nurses, the medical team, and hospital social workers. They are your partners.
- Ask the transplant team to outline the first days, weeks, and months after surgery.
- Keep expectations flexible. Every recovery is unique.

Step 2
Create a Supportive and Safe Home Environment

Bringing your loved one home after a heart transplant is exciting, but it can also be overwhelming. Hospitals are controlled environments with doctors, nurses, and staff watching every detail. At home, you, as the caregiver, are in charge of creating a space where healing can happen.

1. Stay calm if resistance arises; don't take it personally.
2. Encourage the patient gently to follow medical advice.
3. Remind yourself that denial is often part of the healing process.

Because your loved one's immune system is suppressed by anti-rejection medications, your role as caregiver includes maintaining a safe and sanitized environment.

1. Clean frequently touched surfaces, door handles, counters, and remotes.
2. Wash hands often and encourage visitors to do the same.
3. Be honest with family and friends about why visits must be limited.

More About Creating a Supportive and Safe Home Environment

The medications that prevent rejection also weaken the body's defenses. A simple cold can become a serious illness for a heart transplant patient.

- Use phone calls and video chats to help your loved one feel connected.
- Explain to others that this is temporary, and safety must come first.

Beyond medical safety, comfort matters. Your loved one needs a space that is easy to navigate, restful, and filled with things that bring peace.

- Surround them with things that bring encouragement and calm.
- Choose a space with good lighting, fresh air, and easy access to the bathroom.

Step 3
Manage Medications

Managing medications is one of the most important responsibilities of a caregiver. In the beginning, the number of prescriptions can be overwhelming. At first, it may feel like you are running a small pharmacy in your own home. But with time, organization, and patience, this will become routine.

1. Ask the transplant team to explain what each medication does.
2. Know which medications are time-sensitive and must be taken on schedule.
3. Never stop or adjust medications without a doctor's approval.

With so many pills, it's not enough to rely on memory. Having a system is essential for staying on track.

1. Use pill organizers labeled with the days of the week.
2. Keep a written or digital log of dosages and times taken.
3. Have an extra pill organizer filled and ready to go, so when one is finished, the second one is ready for the patient

More About Managing Medications

Your role is not just to hand out pills, but to ensure your loved one is truly protected and cared for in this new life chapter.

- Keep a close eye on refill schedules, especially for anti-rejection medications.
- Take notes at each clinic visit; doctors often adjust prescriptions based on bloodwork.

Anti-rejection medications are powerful; they protect the heart, but they may also affect the rest of the body. As a caregiver, you are in the first line of defense to notice if something is wrong.

- Look for fevers, coughing, or sudden fatigue, and report them immediately to the transplant team.
- Never hesitate to call the doctors if something feels off. Trust your instincts.

Step 4
Attend All Follow-Up Appointments

After a heart transplant, follow-up appointments are essential, especially in the first year. The patient will need frequent appointments to monitor progress, adjust medications, and detect any signs of complications. The caregiver plays a critical role in keeping appointments organized and ensuring that instructions from the medical team are followed.

1. Plan your calendar around these appointments, especially in the first six months.
2. Keep transportation arrangements ready, as patients can't drive for the first six months.
3. Remind yourself that appointment frequency will decrease with time.

Doctors often share complex instructions during visits. Having the caregiver present ensures that nothing gets lost or forgotten.

1. Take notes during every appointment.
2. Ask follow-up questions to clarify instructions.
3. Repeat information back to doctors to confirm accuracy.

More About Attending All Follow-up Appointments

Sometimes at the beginning, bloodwork or symptoms will prompt urgent appointments, or even hospital readmission. While unsettling, these visits are part of the process and should be handled quickly and calmly.

- Always answer calls from the transplant clinic promptly.
- Keep a bag packed with essentials in case of an unexpected hospital stay.

The first months of caregiving can feel like a full-time job. Doctors may change medication often based on bloodwork, which at first will seem overwhelming.

- Be patient with the process; progress is gradual.
- View follow-up visits as reassurance rather than inconvenience.

Step 5
Monitor for Signs of Infection or Rejection

After a transplant, the patient's greatest risk is serious infection or organ rejection. Both can happen suddenly, and both require immediate medical attention. The caregiver's role is to observe closely and act quickly if something is wrong.

1. Vigilance, consistency, and communication with your medical team make all the difference.
2. Even with medication, the body may attempt to reject the new heart. Warning signs can appear in subtle ways, so caregivers must stay alert.
3. Keep a log of changes to share with the medical team. Report any changes to the transplant medical team promptly. Anti-Rejection drugs suppress the immune system, leaving the patient vulnerable.
4. Watch for signs of chills, cough, or sore throat. Avoid contact with anyone who is sick, even with mild symptoms.
5. Monitor incision sites for redness, swelling, or drainage.

More About Monitoring for Signs of Infection or Rejection

When the patient first comes home, isolation and rest are critical. Visitors should be limited, especially in the first weeks and months.

- Encourage virtual visits until the medical team says that in-person visits are safe.
- Understand that infection and rejection risks decrease over time but remain lifelong concerns.

Monitoring for signs of infection or rejection may feel like walking on a tightrope at first. Caregivers may find themselves constantly watching, worrying, and second-guessing.

- Over time, vigilance becomes part of the routine.
- With each clear check-up, confidence grows. Staying alert and trusting the process gives both the caregiver and the patient the reassurance to move forward with hope.

Step 6
Encourage a Heart-Healthy Lifestyle

A heart transplant gives a patient a second chance at life, but protecting that gift takes commitment to healthy living.

1. Diet, exercise, and daily habits play a huge role in long-term success.
2. Avoid processed foods, fried foods, and excess salt.
3. Follow the exercise program outlined by the transplant team.

Beyond diet and exercise, daily routines matter. Rest, hydration, and avoiding harmful habits all play a part in keeping the new heart strong.

1. Ensure the patient gets enough sleep.
2. Encourage drinking plenty of water throughout the day.
3. Avoid alcohol, smoking, or unhealthy coping habits.

More About Encouraging a Heart-Healthy Lifestyle

Doctors often say that a heart transplant can add decades to a patient's life *if* they take care of their new heart.

- Small, consistent choices lead to long-term health.
- A heart-healthy lifestyle benefits the caregiver as well as the patient

Healthy living is easier when done together. The caregiver can set the tone by adopting the same habits, making it a team effort rather than a burden on the patient.

- Cook and eat the same meals together.
- Join in on daily walks or light exercise.

Step 7
Provide Emotional Support

Recovery after a heart transplant is not only physical, it's deeply emotional. Patients often feel a wide range of feelings, from relief and gratitude to anxiety, depression, or guilt.

1. As a caregiver, your role is to support them through these ups and downs.
2. Utilize patience, compassion, and understanding.
3. Emotional healing is just as important as physical healing in the transplant journey.

Sometimes the most powerful form of support is simply listening. Patients may express fear, frustration, or even guilt about receiving an organ. Caregivers who listen with empathy help ease these heavy emotions.

1. Give your full attention during conversations.
2. Allow them to share without trying to fix everything.
3. Use encouraging words to remind them they are not alone. Sometimes, just quietly sitting with the patient gives them reassurance.

More About Providing Emotional Support

Emotional healing is a process that unfolds over time. Caregivers can provide steady encouragement and create a safe space for emotions to be expressed.

- With support, patients often move from fear to gratitude, and from uncertainty to confidence.
- Remind the patient that receiving an organ is a gift, not a burden.

Providing emotional support means standing beside someone in their darkest moments as well as their brightest. It requires compassion, patience, and resilience. This step reminds us that recovery is not only about the heart; it is also about the spirit.

- Patience and presence matter more than perfect words.
- Emotional support helps strengthen both the patient and the caregiver.

Step 8
Take Care of Yourself

Caregiving after a transplant is demanding, both physically and emotionally. Many caregivers focus so much on the patient that they forget their own needs. The caregiver's health directly impacts their ability to provide support. Taking care of yourself is not selfish—it's necessary.

1. Set aside time to rest, even in small moments.
2. Make sure to eat balanced meals and stay hydrated.
3. Spend a few moments outdoors now and then for fresh air and sunlight.

Caregivers often put themselves last. Preserving your own health ensures you can continue to provide strength and stability for the patient. A caregiver who is cared for becomes a stronger caregiver.

1. Caring for yourself sets an example for the patient as well.
2. Small acts of self-care add up to big differences in resilience.

More About Taking Care of Yourself

Taking care of yourself may seem difficult when you're focused on the patient and their care, but it is vital. Healthy caregivers are better able to manage stress, provide emotional stability, and handle themselves calmly in emergencies.

- Consider journaling to release your emotions and track your journey.
- Practice deep breathing or relaxation exercises.

Simple intentional practices can restore your energy and bring calm in the midst of challenges.

- Engage in light exercise, such as walking to lift your mood.
- Share your experiences with a trusted friend or counselor.

Step 9
Know the Signs of Caregiver Burnout

Caregiving for a heart transplant patient is rewarding but can also be extremely demanding. The combination of strict medication schedules, transplant follow-up appointments, infection control routines, and emotional support can leave caregivers exhausted. Recognizing burnout early is essential. It not only affects the caregiver's health but also the patient's safety.

1. Be prepared for a high level of responsibility.
2. Caregiving for a heart transplant patient will feel overwhelming, especially in the first 6 months to a year.
3. Remember, a caregiver's health can directly impact a patient's health.

Burnout can show up in many ways. Caregivers may feel overwhelmed by constant demands and restrictions, especially since the patient's life depends on support.

1. Watch for mood swings, resentment, or loss of patience.
2. Notice physical signs such as headaches, fatigue, or sleep problems.
3. Pay attention to feelings of isolation or hopelessness.

More About Knowing the Signs of Caregiver Burnout

Recognizing burnout is only the first step. Caregivers must also take action to protect their well-being before exhaustion leads to mistakes or illness.

- Ask trusted friends or family to help with meals, errands, or household chores.
- Schedule short breaks, even if only for a short walk or quiet time.

Burnout is one of the hidden challenges of heart transplant caregiving. The strict routines and the weight of responsibility can leave caregivers depleted. Recognizing the signs early and taking steps to rest and recharge makes it possible to keep going.

- Burnout doesn't mean failure; it means you need support.
- Delegating responsibilities strengthens caregiving; it doesn't weaken it.

Step 10
Celebrate Milestones

The transplant journey is long and demanding, but it is also filled with moments of progress worth celebrating. Milestones remind both patient and caregiver that the effort is paying off, and that recovery, while slow, is moving forward.

1. Recognizing these achievements builds confidence.
2. Celebrating each milestone renews hope.
3. Milestone celebrations strengthen the bond between patient and caregiver.

At first, the transplant patient will attend weekly follow-up appointments. Over time, visits may change to every two weeks, then every month, and eventually once a year, depending on their bloodwork results.

1. Mark all the milestone changes on the calendar.
2. Acknowledge the progress with encouraging words.
3. Use the extra time as an opportunity to enjoy something special together.

More About Celebrating Milestones

Over time, restrictions will ease. Travel, dining out, and gathering with family and friends will become possible again. These moments are worth celebrating as signs of returning to everyday life.

- Plan a special outing when the medical team approves.
- Reintroduce favorite activities slowly and safely.

Recovery from a heart transplant is often measured in small steps, not giant leaps. Every milestone, big or small, is a sign of moving closer to normal life.

- Encourage independence while staying watchful.
- Share these victories with supportive friends or family.

Step 11
Don't Be Afraid of Change

At first, the patient will rely completely on the caregiver. Within months, they may begin to resume their independence. This transition can feel strange for caregivers who have been constantly needed.

1. Understand that independence is a sign of healing, not rejection of your role.
2. Encourage progress even when it feels hard to step back.
3. Allow the patient to take small steps of independence safely.

Prepare for changes in activities. Restrictions around travel, driving, or socializing will gradually ease as the patient gets stronger.

1. Follow the medical team's guidance about resuming safe activities.
2. Encourage reentry into daily life gradually.

More About Don't Be Afraid of Change

Embrace your evolving role as caregiver. Change can be unsettling, but it is a natural part of recovery. Each change, whether in medication, daily life, or appointments, reflects progress. The caregiver's ability to adapt ensures that the patient moves forward with confidence.

- Change is a sign of growth and healing.
- Independence is the goal, not a threat.

Adapting to change is one of the caregiver's greatest challenges. What once felt essential, such as constant presence and strict routines, gradually shift as the patient heals.

- Take pride in how far you and the patient have come together.
- Recognize that letting go is a normal part of healing.

Step 12
Getting Stronger

With time, patience, and careful management, the heart transplant patient begins to regain strength. This part of the journey is often the most rewarding, as progress becomes more visible and daily life feels less fragile.

1. The challenge shifts from constant protection to encouraging independence.
2. Reevaluate daily tasks and hand more responsibility back to the patient.
3. Take pride in how much both of you have accomplished.

By this stage, many caregivers notice a rhythm. As medical demands start to decrease, the patient shows resilience, and routines become more manageable. The hard work is paying off.

1. This step in the journey offers hope and reassurance.
2. This stage proves that healing is possible and the new heart is doing its job.
3. Strength for the patient means strength for you, the caregiver.

More About Getting Stronger

Activity increases as the patient's strength builds. Walking or light activity may be encouraged by the medical team.

- Monitor for signs of fatigue or over-exertion.
- Support gradual increases in activity.

Caregivers may feel conflicted as patients begin to do more for themselves. While it may be hard to stop being so protective and start letting go, independence is what the patient is striving for.

- Provide oversight without microman-aging.
- Encourage confidence in their ability to care for themselves.

Step 13
Returning to Everyday Life

After months of strict routine, limited contact, and constant medical oversight, life gradually begins to feel normal again. While normal may look different from what it did before the transplant, returning to everyday life is worth celebrating.

1. As strength returns, many heart transplant recipients can return to work or resume household responsibilities.
2. Encourage pacing and increase gradually.
3. Help balance rest with responsibility.

Reintroduce social activities and travel. With medical approval, patients may begin to travel, attend social gatherings, and enjoy activities outside the home.

1. Reintroduce meaningful traditions or family activities.
2. Celebrate the return of small pleasures, like dining out or attending events.
3. Practice ongoing gratitude. Acknowledge the gift of life that made this stage possible.

More About Returning to Everyday Life

Returning to everyday life is also a time of reflection. Patient and caregiver alike may feel deep gratitude toward the donor, the medical team, and each other.

- Consider supporting donor awareness or transplant organizations as a way of giving back and honoring the organ donor.
- Express gratitude often, in words or actions

Everyday life now may not look identical to life before, but it offers a chance to create a new normal. Part of that new normal is a deep sense of gratitude for a second chance at life, for the donor who made this possible, and for being able to continue celebrating life with your loved one.

- Normal will feel like a celebration of life because it is.
- Life will feel less like survival and more like living again.

Step 14
Evaluating Your Situation

Caregiving for a heart transplant patient is a long-term commitment. Over time, the demands may shift, but the responsibility remains.

1. The heart transplant patient will remain on rejection medication for life.
2. Be responsible for constant medication refills and making sure the patient has taken all pills every day.
3. Medications are always included in the patient's travel bag whenever traveling away from home.

Heart transplant caregiving is a marathon, not a sprint; it requires planning for the long haul.

1. A few adjustments that need to be made in the life of a heart transplant patient are part of the new normal.
2. Stay in periodic contact with the heart transplant team.
3. Make sure the patient is aware of and attends all follow-up appointments, which will be fewer but will be for life.
4. Start enjoying life again.

More About Evaluating Your Situation

You can now release the constant vigilance and relax more. You will find that the patient has begun to be less like your patient and more like your loved one again. It's time to celebrate.

- Recognize that the patient is stronger and more capable now.
- Allow confidence to replace constant worry.

Over time, the patient will want to manage more of their own care. It's normal for caregivers to feel uneasy at first, but trust grows as stability builds.

- Gradually reduce the intensity of your oversight.
- Accept that independence is a sign of success, not loss.

Step 15
Don't Be Afraid to Let Go

After months of constant care, watchfulness, and responsibility, one of the hardest tasks is learning to let go. At first, it may feel unnatural after being so involved in every detail, yet letting go is essential to allow the patient to reclaim their independence and their life

1. Encourage the patient to manage medications with supervision.
2. Acknowledge that your role is changing, not disappearing.
3. Create new goals and routines for your own life.

Caregiving may have consumed every part of your life. As your loved one becomes more independent, it's important to rediscover yourself and balance in your own life

1. Reconnect with hobbies, work, or friendships.
2. Balance supporting your loved one with honoring your own needs.
3. Embrace life again with strength, gratitude, and new purpose.

More About Don't Be Afraid to Let Go

The final step of a heart transplant caregiver's journey is acceptance. Accept that your loved one has grown strong, and the gift of life is being fully lived. Letting go does not diminish the love, sacrifice, or importance of caregiving; letting go honors it.

- Caregivers remain important even as their role shifts.
- Letting go allows both patient and caregiver to move forward with freedom and hope.

Final thoughts: Caring for a heart trans-plant recipient is one of the greatest responsibilities a loved one can face. It is a journey of challenges, adjustments, and moments of deep uncertainty. And yet, it is also a journey marked by courage, resilience, and the incredible gift of life itself.

- There will be moments when you feel exhausted, unsure, or even overwhelmed, but there will also be moments of great joy.
- Finally, never forget that you are not alone. And above all, the strength you need for this journey is already within you.

You've finished. Before you go …

Post/Share that you finished this book.

Please star-rate this book.

Reviews are solid gold to writers. Please take a few minutes to give us some itty bitty feedback.

ABOUT THE AUTHOR

Luann Owens is a caregiver, speaker, and storyteller whose life was forever changed the day her husband, Coach Jimmy Owens, was told his heart was failing and he would need a transplant to survive. What began as a marriage rooted in love, faith, and shared purpose quickly became a journey through hospital hallways, ICU rooms, long waiting nights, and whispered prayers. Luann did not choose the role of caregiver, but she embraced it with courage, compassion, and unwavering devotion.

For more than two decades, Luann has stood beside Jimmy as his partner in life, faith, and mission. When his health crisis turned their world upside down, she became his advocate, his protector, his encourager, and his steady hand through the most uncertain days. From the moment he was placed on lifesupport to the miracle of receiving a new heart, Luann walked every step with him, learning, growing, and discovering a strength she never knew she had.

With a voice that blends honesty, humor, faith, and compassion, Luann speaks to caregivers as one of them. She believes caregiving is a sacred calling one that deserves support, recognition, and grace. Her mission is to help caregivers feel seen, strengthened, and empowered as they walk one of the most important journeys of their lives.

If you enjoyed this Itty Bitty™ book, you might also like…

- **Your Amazing Itty Bitty™ Self Care For Caregivers Book** by Janie Becker
- **Your Amazing Itty Bitty™ Book Of Faith** by Kelly D. Smith
- **Your Amazing Itty Bitty™ Healing In Ways You Never Thought Possible Book** by Dr. Dolores Fazzino, DNP

Or any of the many Amazing Itty Bitty™ books available online at www.ittybittypublishing.com

www.ingramcontent.com/pod-product-compliance
Lightning Source LLC
Chambersburg PA
CBHW072244240926
51846CB00012B/612
* 9 7 8 1 9 5 9 9 6 4 6 3 6 *